HERBAL REMEDIES FOR DEPRESSION

Empowering Your Mind Naturally For Embracing Botanical Solutions, Nurturing Mental Resilience, Optimal Well-Being, And Brain Healing

DR. CARDEN KYRIE

DISCLAIMER

The only goal of this book is informational. Every effort has been taken by the author and publisher to ensure that the information provided is accurate. But the material in this book is given "as is," without any express or implied representation, warranty, or condition as to its accuracy, completeness, or suitability for any particular purpose.

Any loss, damage, or injury resulting from using the information in this book, or from any action or decision made as a result of such use, will not be covered by the author's or publisher's liability. It is recommended that readers seek the assistance of a certified specialist for guidance specific to their situation.

The opinions and viewpoints conveyed in this book belong to the author and may not necessarily represent the official stance or policies of any specified organizations or people. Any likeness to real-life occurrences, places, or people—living or deceased—is wholly coincidental.

No specific product, service, or therapy discussed in this book is endorsed by the author or publisher. Any reference to goods or services is made only for informative reasons and is not intended as a recommendation or endorsement.

Before making any judgments or acting on any information, readers are urged to independently confirm it all. Any unfavorable effects or repercussions arising from the usage of the material included in this book are disclaimed by the author and publisher.

By using this book, you consent to absolving the publisher and author of any and all claims, obligations, or losses resulting from your use of the material in it.

I appreciate your cooperation and understanding.

TABLE OF CONTENTS

CHAPTER ONE

INTRODUCTION TO DEPRESSION

TYPES AND DEFINITIONS OF DEPRESSION

A complicated and multidimensional mental health condition that affects millions of people globally is depression. It is typified by enduring depressive and dismal feelings as well as a lack of interest in or enjoyment from once-enjoyed activities. Depression affects more than just the emotional sphere; it also has an impact on a person's relationships, career, and general well-being.

Depression comes in a variety of forms, each with its symptoms and traits. One of the most prevalent types is Major Depressive Disorder (MDD), which is characterized by a persistently depressed mood, exhaustion, irregular sleep patterns, and a decreased capacity for concentration. Dysthymia, another name for persistent depression disorder (PDD), is characterized by persistent but milder symptoms that might persist for years. Manic-depressive illness, which was once known as bipolar disorder, was defined by recurrent episodes of depression and mania or hypomania. Seasonal affective disorder (SAD), postpartum depression, and atypical depression are among the several kinds that might cause distinct difficulties for individuals afflicted.

FREQUENCY AND EFFECT

Depression is a major public health concern due to its startling frequency. The World Health Organization (WHO) estimates that depression affects over 264 million people globally. This mental health disorder affects people from all areas of life and does not discriminate based on age, gender, or socioeconomic background. Depression has a significant negative influence on sufferers as well as their families, communities, and society at large.

Numerous negative effects, both psychological and physical, can result from depression. Depression frequently results in cognitive impairment, which makes it difficult for depressed people to concentrate on tasks and make judgments. Many people experience sleep disorders, such as insomnia or oversleeping. Changes in energy and appetite are examples of physical symptoms that can coexist with the emotional aspects of depression. Depression has a profound effect on social interactions because depressed people tend to isolate themselves from friends and family, which exacerbates feelings of loneliness.

Depression at work can lead to lower output and absenteeism, which has a larger negative impact on economic productivity. Depression affects healthcare systems as well since the expense of care and treatment puts pressure on available resources. The worldwide consequences of depression underscore the necessity for heightened consciousness, prompt identification, and efficacious remedial measures.

Comprehending the various expressions of depression and recognizing its extensive occurrence are essential measures in establishing a more sympathetic and encouraging community. Developing all-encompassing strategies for the prevention, management, and treatment of depression is made feasible by considering the intricate interactions between biological, psychological, and environmental components. In the end, reducing the effects of depression on people and communities will need teamwork and the development of a mental health and well-being-focused culture.

CHAPTER TWO

DEPRESSION'S CAUSES

BIOLOGICAL CIRCUMSTANCES

Although depression is a complicated mental illness influenced by many different circumstances, biological factors are crucial to its beginning and progression. One such element is genetic predisposition; studies indicate that people with a family history of depression may be more prone to the condition. Unbalances in neurotransmitters can contribute to the biochemical basis of depression.

Neurotransmitter levels, including those of serotonin, norepinephrine, and dopamine, can fluctuate, interfering with brain cell communication and affecting mood control. Furthermore, depression has been connected to anatomical abnormalities in the brain, especially in regions related to emotion processing and control.

PSYCHOLOGICAL VARIABLES

awareness of the intricacy of depression requires an awareness of the interplay of psychological variables in its appearance. Common psychological contributions include maladaptive coping mechanisms, negative thought patterns, and cognitive distortions. People who have a gloomy outlook on the world could see things negatively, which would feed a vicious cycle of negative thinking. Depression susceptibility is also influenced by certain personality features, such as high degrees of neuroticism.

Especially in childhood, traumatic life experiences can mold cognitive schemas and promote the emergence of depressive tendencies. Chronic stress, whether it is from relationships, the workplace, or personal struggles, can also weaken a person's psychological resilience and hasten the onset of depression.

ENVIRONMENTAL FACTORS

The onset and worsening of depression are significantly influenced by environmental factors. Depression risk is correlated with socioeconomic conditions like unemployment and poverty.

Depressive episodes can be triggered by stressful life events including divorce, the death of a loved one, or unstable finances. Depression risk is also influenced by environmental variables such as social isolation and a lack of social support.

Furthermore, an individual's sense of achievement and self-worth can be shaped by cultural influences and societal expectations, which might impact the onset of depression symptoms. Because alcohol and drugs can be abused and utilized as maladaptive coping techniques, substance addiction can exacerbate the link between environmental variables and depression.

Developing thorough treatment strategies requires an understanding of depression as a complex disorder comprising biological, psychological, and environmental aspects. Incorporating interventions that target these different characteristics can improve therapeutic strategies' efficacy and advance a more comprehensive knowledge of the condition.

CHAPTER THREE

TRADITIONAL DEPRESSION TREATMENTS DRUGS

In the traditional treatment of depression, medications are essential, and prescriptions for various drug classes are frequently given to reduce symptoms. Antidepressants are often used, including tricyclic antidepressants (TCAs), serotonin-norepinephrine reuptake inhibitors (SNRIs), and selective serotonin reuptake inhibitors (SSRIs). While SNRIs, like venlafaxine, target both serotonin and norepinephrine, SSRIs, like fluoxetine and sertraline, function by raising serotonin levels in the brain. Amitriptyline is one example of a tricyclic antidepressant that affects several neurotransmitters. By regulating neurotransmitter levels, these drugs seek to rectify the chemical abnormalities linked to depression.

Antidepressant efficacy varies from person to person, and selecting the appropriate drug frequently necessitates some trial and error. Furthermore, it could take a few weeks to experience the complete therapeutic benefits. Common side effects include nausea, sleeplessness, and erectile dysfunction. Notwithstanding these difficulties, drugs continue to be a vital component in the treatment of depression, offering many people relief.

PSYCHOANALYSIS

Talk therapy, often known as psychotherapy, is another essential part of traditional depression treatment. There are several types of psychotherapy used, the most popular being cognitive-behavioral treatment (CBT). Cognitive Behavioral Therapy (CBT) aims to recognize and address the negative thought patterns and behaviors that underlie depressive symptoms. It gives people the coping mechanisms and abilities they need to control their stress and enhance their general mental health.

Other types of psychotherapy include interpersonal therapy, which deals with relationship problems, and psychodynamic therapy, which investigates unconscious patterns and unresolved conflicts. The therapeutic alliance itself can play a critical role in the effectiveness of psychotherapy by giving patients a safe, accepting environment in which to disclose their feelings. The best results are frequently obtained when psychotherapy and medicine are combined, providing a comprehensive approach to treating depression.

ELECTROSHOCK TREATMENT

More intrusive and intense than other forms of treatment, electroconvulsive therapy (ECT) is usually used in cases of acutely dangerous severe depression or when other therapies have failed. With electrical brain stimulation, controlled seizures are induced during ECT. It is thought that the seizure activity alters neurotransmitter release and receptor sensitivity, while the precise mechanisms are not entirely understood.

To reduce discomfort, ECT is frequently given while under general anesthesia, and a course of treatment typically entails several sessions. Even though ECT works well, there are certain negative effects to be aware of, such as confusion and short-term memory loss just after treatment. When deciding whether to pursue ECT, one carefully considers the advantages and disadvantages of the procedure. It is typically saved for particular situations where a quick and noticeable improvement is required, including in the case of severe depressive episodes or when other therapies have failed.

Traditional therapies for depression involve a variety of techniques, including medication, psychotherapy, and, in certain situations, electroconvulsive therapy. Combining these modalities enables a customized strategy that takes into account the various requirements and preferences of people who are struggling with depression. It emphasizes how crucial it is for patients and medical providers to work together to negotiate the complexity of depression and achieve long-term recovery.

CHAPTER FOUR

A COMPREHENSIVE STRATEGY FOR MENTAL HEALTH

MIND-BODY LINK

Recognizing the indisputable link between mental and physical well-being, the holistic approach to mental health stresses the complex interactions between the mind and body. This method's cornerstone is the mind-body connection, which holds that physical and mental health are interdependent and that mental health cannot exist without the other. Comprehending and tackling this interdependence is essential to promoting overall mental health.

FACTORS RELATED TO LIFESTYLE

The way of life has a significant impact on how mental health results turn out. A holistic approach recognizes that everyday routines, habits, and lifestyle choices have an impact on mental health. Good lifestyle decisions, such as consistent exercise, enough sleep, and stress reduction, greatly support a resilient and balanced mind. The body's natural mood enhancers, endorphins, are released when you exercise, for example, demonstrating the mutually beneficial relationship between physical and mental wellness.

DIETARY TACTICS

Another crucial element of the holistic approach to mental health is nutritional interventions. It is impossible to exaggerate the role nutrition plays in mental wellness. Neurotransmitter activity and brain function are directly impacted by the food we eat. Emotional stability and maximum cognitive function depend on a diet high in vital nutrients. Foods high in nutrients give the building blocks needed for the production of neurotransmitters, which affect mood, thinking, and mental health in general.

DIET IS IMPORTANT FOR MENTAL HEALTH

In the context of dietary tactics, meals that elevate mood receive particular attention. Certain meals have been found to have the ability to improve mental health and mood. For instance, omega-3 fatty acids, which are present in fatty fish, have been linked to a decrease in depressive symptoms. Rich in folate, dark leafy greens have also been connected to happier moods. Incorporating these nutrients into the diet to enhance mental health physiologically is encouraged by the holistic approach.

CRUCIAL ELEMENTS FOR HEALTHY BRAIN FUNCTION

Within the holistic framework, essential nutrients for brain health are important factors to take into account. Antioxidants, vitamins, minerals, omega-3 fatty acids, and other nutrients are essential for preserving cognitive function and preventing mental health issues. For example, the synthesis of neurotransmitters depends on the vitamin B complex, and antioxidants shield the brain from oxidative damage. Therefore, maintaining a healthy brain and, consequently, fostering mental well-being requires a diet that is both well-balanced and nutrient-rich.

The holistic approach to mental health includes a thorough comprehension of the relationship between the mind and body, the influence of lifestyle variables, and the importance of nutritional approaches. Understanding the role nutrition plays in mental health highlights the necessity of a comprehensive and nourishing approach to promote mental and physical well-being. People can empower themselves to develop resilience and improve their general quality of life by adopting this comprehensive viewpoint.

CHAPTER FIVE

HERBAL DEPRESSION TREATMENTS
AN OVERVIEW OF HERBAL MEDICINE

Herbal medicine is a holistic approach to healing that uses plants and plant extracts to improve health and treat a variety of illnesses. It is sometimes referred to as phytotherapy or botanical medicine. With roots in ancient medical systems like Ayurveda, Traditional Chinese Medicine (TCM), and Native American healing customs, this technique has been around for centuries. Using plants' therapeutic qualities to enhance the body's healing processes is the core idea of herbal therapy.

The wide range of bioactive substances found in herbs, such as terpenes, flavonoids, alkaloids, and essential oils, are what give them their therapeutic qualities. Herbal remedies can be administered in a variety of ways depending on the patient's preferences and medical conditions because they are frequently made as teas, tinctures, capsules, or salves. It is significant to remember that, even though herbal medicine may have advantages, speaking with a healthcare provider is always advisable, particularly for people who already have medical issues or are on other medications.

PARTICULAR HERBS AND THEIR ADVANTAGES

1. Hypericum perforatum, sometimes known as St. John's Wort: One of the most well-known herbs for treating mild to moderate depression is probably this one. Its main ingredients, including hypericin and hyperforin, are thought to affect neurotransmitters that are important for mood control, such as serotonin. Studies indicate that St. John's Wort may be just as useful in treating depression in some situations as some traditional antidepressants. It should be used with caution though, as it may interfere with other drugs.

2. Ginkgo biloba: Known for improving cognition, ginkgo biloba is frequently included in herbal depression

therapies. The herb's uplifting effects on mood might be attributed to its blood circulation-boosting and antioxidant properties. Some research suggests that ginkgo biloba may help reduce depressive symptoms, but more trials are required to confirm its effectiveness.

3. Lavender (Lavandula spp.): Often linked to calmness and alleviation of tension, lavender may help with the symptoms of anxiety and depression. The nervous system may be calmed by the aromatic chemicals in lavender oil, such as linalyl acetate and linalool. Relaxation and mental health may be enhanced by adding lavender to aromatherapy or applying lavender oil to massage therapy.

4. Rhodiola Rosea: Known as an adaptogenic plant, Rhodiola Rosea is effective in assisting the body in adjusting to stress. It might help maintain the proper levels of neurotransmitters like dopamine and serotonin, which would enhance mood and increase resistance to stress. Although studies on the antidepressant effects of Rhodiola are encouraging, further research is required

to completely comprehend the processes and efficacy of this herb.

5. Withania somnifera, sometimes known as ashwagandha, is a well-known herb in Ayurvedic medicine. It is an adaptogen, meaning it helps the body cope with stress. The active ingredients in it, known as withanolides, have the potential to affect neurotransmitters and the HPA axis, which is involved in the stress response. According to certain research, ashwagandha may be able to help manage mood disorders by lowering anxiety and acting as an antidepressant.

A variety of plants, each with its collection of bioactive components and possible advantages, are used in herbal treatments for depression. Although some herbs have the potential to promote mental health, it is important to take caution when using them and seek advice from medical professionals to ensure safety and effectiveness in specific instances.

CHAPTER SIX

MIND-BODY TECHNIQUES

MEDITATION AND MINDFULNESS

Both of these age-old, contemplative traditions-based techniques are becoming increasingly well-known in today's wellness discourse. Meditation is the practice of using different techniques, including breath awareness or mantra repetition, to cultivate a focused and peaceful state of mind. Conversely, mindfulness places a strong emphasis on being present in the here and now and objectively monitoring thoughts and sensations.

The aim of both activities is the same: to promote emotional equilibrium, mental clarity, and increased awareness. Regular mindfulness and meditation have been linked to improved attention, lower stress levels, and improved mental health overall, according to research.

YOGA FOR MENTAL WELL-BEING

Yoga is an age-old Indian discipline that has developed into a comprehensive strategy for both physical and mental wellness. Beyond its physical asanas or postures, yoga also combines meditation and breath control. This comprehensive strategy is thought to improve mental health by encouraging rest and lowering stress. The incorporation of mindfulness into yoga promotes a sense of inner calm by encouraging practitioners to establish connections with their bodies and thoughts. Studies have shown that yoga, which combines mindfulness with physical exercise in a special way, can be a useful adjunctive treatment for several mental health issues, including anxiety and depression.

Qigong and Tai Chi are mind-body exercises with slow, flowing motions and concentrated breathing. They have their roots in Chinese martial arts and traditional medicine. The goal of these exercises is to develop the body's "qi," or life force. Beyond their health benefits, Qigong and Tai Chi are linked to better mental health.

The focus on breath awareness and mindful movement promotes balance and tranquility while lowering tension and anxiety. Research indicates that consistent practice of Qigong and Tai Chi may improve mental health, including improved emotional stability and cognitive function.

DEPRESSION AND PHYSICAL EXERCISE

There has been a lot of discussion on the connection between mental health and physical exercise, especially in the setting of depression. Regular exercise has been demonstrated to have antidepressant effects by affecting neurotransmitter levels and encouraging the release of endorphins, which are the body's natural mood enhancers. Moreover, exercise promotes better sleep hygiene, higher self-esteem, and a feeling of achievement. Structured exercise regimens are becoming more widely acknowledged as an effective therapeutic approach to alleviate depression, akin to conventional interventions like psychotherapy and medication.

THE RELATIONSHIP BETWEEN MOOD AND EXERCISE

Exercise and mood control are related in a complicated way by physiological, psychological, and neurobiological variables interacting. Serotonin and dopamine are two neurotransmitters that are released during physical activity and are essential for mood control. Exercise also increases brain connection and encourages the development of new neurons, which benefits emotional and cognitive health. It's clear that exercise, whether it be yoga, strength training, or aerobics, improves mood. Frequent exercise maintains general mental resilience and prevents anxiety and depression symptoms in addition to relieving them.

DEVELOPING AN EXERCISE PROGRAM

One of the most important things you can do to support your physical and emotional health is to create and stick to an exercise program. To ensure sustainability, the first step is to select activities that fit with personal tastes and objectives. Establishing attainable goals increases motivation by fostering a sense of success. Including variation in the routine keeps things interesting and avoids boredom. Overall fitness is also enhanced by striking a balance between strength training, flexibility training, and aerobic exercise. The advantages of exercise for mental health can be amplified by adding mindfulness practices, such as paying attention to breath and movement. Being consistent is crucial, and building a fun and long-lasting habit that benefits the body and mind may be accomplished through slow and steady improvement.

CHAPTER SEVEN

MODIFICATIONS TO LIFESTYLE FOR MENTAL HEALTH

DEPRESSION AND SLEEP

Sleep is essential for mental health, and there is a particularly significant link between sleep and depression. Several research works have demonstrated a reciprocal association between depression and sleep, whereby depression can interfere with regular sleep patterns and sleep quality can lead to the onset or worsening of depressive symptoms. It is impossible to exaggerate the significance of getting enough sleep for preserving mental wellness. For mental clarity, emotional stability, and general stress resilience, one must get enough good sleep.

THE VALUE OF GOOD SLEEP

It's essential to practice good sleep hygiene if you want to get good sleep. Establishing routines and setting up the environment for comfortable sleep is part of sleep hygiene. A regular sleep schedule, a cozy sleeping environment, avoiding stimulants like caffeine close to bedtime, and using relaxation techniques before bed are some important sleep hygiene recommendations. Through the promotion of emotional stability and cognitive clarity, these techniques can have a substantial positive impact on mental health in addition to improving sleep quality.

STRESS REDUCTION

Reducing stress is yet another essential component of preserving mental health. Crucial actions in this process include recognizing and dealing with stressors. It entails identifying the elements that lead to stress, be they conflict inside oneself or outside demands, or both. Upon identification, measures for managing stress can be put into practice. This could involve time management, problem-solving skills, realistic goal-setting, and the ability to adjust to unforeseen difficulties.

In terms of mental health, proactive stress management lowers the possibility that stressors will result in more severe mental health problems.

TECHNIQUES FOR RELAXATION

Relaxation methods are effective strategies for preserving mental equilibrium in addition to managing stress. Incorporating techniques like progressive muscle relaxation, mindfulness meditation, and deep breathing exercises can help lower stress levels, ease anxiety, and enhance mental health in general. These methods help people feel more at ease and empower them to deal with the difficulties they face daily.

SOCIAL INTERACTION

A basic human need, social interaction has a significant impact on mental health. Developing and maintaining relationships is a major factor in emotional resilience. Strong bonds with friends, family, and a larger social network offer a safety net that helps counteract the damaging impacts of stress and misfortune. Social connections facilitate emotional expression, empathy, and the sharing of experiences, all of which contribute to a person's feeling of emotional stability and belonging.

ASSISTIVE SYSTEMS

Building strong support networks is essential to preserving mental health. Building a network of people who can provide understanding, practical help, and emotional support during trying times is crucial. This could entail getting in touch with loved ones, friends, or mental health specialists. A willingness to ask for assistance when necessary and open communication are essential elements of creating support networks that work.

Modifying one's lifestyle can significantly improve mental health. It is crucial to pay close attention to factors like social interactions, stress management, and sleep.

CHAPTER EIGHT

COMBINING CONVENTIONAL CARE WITH NATURAL SOLUTIONS

A cooperative approach that acknowledges the benefits of both conventional and alternative medical procedures is necessary to integrate natural therapies with treatment. To give patients full, all-encompassing care, this teamwork is crucial. Healthcare providers, such as physicians, nurses, and practitioners of complementary and alternative medicine, can collaborate to develop treatment programs that are tailored to each patient's specific needs.

WORKING TOGETHER

A collaborative approach recognizes that many treatment approaches have unique advantages and disadvantages. While natural therapies may help with long-term well-being and preventive measures, conventional medicine frequently shines in acute care and crisis management. Healthcare professionals can give patients with a more customized and varied variety of treatment alternatives by merging the advantages of both strategies.

COLLABORATING WITH MEDICAL PROFESSIONALS

Collaboration with medical specialists is essential to a successful integration. Mutual respect, open communication, and an awareness of one another's areas of competence are necessary for this kind of cooperation. To improve the general standard of patient care, conventional medical professionals and providers of alternative medicine can exchange information, research results, and clinical experiences. Practitioners can gain a more sophisticated understanding of the numerous elements driving health outcomes by working together across disciplinary boundaries.

SHARING TREATMENT OPTIONS

To guarantee that patients are knowledgeable and actively involved in their healthcare decisions, effective treatment choice communication is essential. Patients and healthcare professionals should have candid conversations regarding the possible advantages and disadvantages of both conventional and natural treatments. As a result, patients are more equipped to make decisions based on their preferences, values, and overall health objectives. To improve treatment adherence overall and build a solid patient-provider relationship, shared decision-making becomes essential.

Furthermore, healthcare providers must be aware of the range of alternative medicines available to include natural cures with conventional treatment. This covers, among other things, nutritional supplements, acupuncture, chiropractic adjustments, and herbal medicine. Healthcare professionals can make well-informed recommendations by having a thorough grasp of these medicines and taking into account their potential interactions and compatibility with traditional treatments.

Healthcare practitioners also need to receive continual education and training to integrate natural therapies into conventional care. Keeping up with the most recent findings, safety precautions, and evidence-based procedures guarantees that healthcare professionals can administer the most modern and efficient integrative therapies. This dedication to lifelong learning makes it possible to provide patient-centered, high-quality care that keeps up with changing medical standards.

A cooperative strategy based on honest communication and a shared dedication to the health of the patient is the most effective way to include natural therapies with conventional treatment. When medical experts collaborate, they can take advantage of the advantages of both techniques to offer a more thorough and individualized treatment plan.

www.ingramcontent.com/pod-product-compliance
Lightning Source LLC
Chambersburg PA
CBHW060849260726
48661CB00002B/692